EVERYTHING ABOUT

HCG DIET

Complete Nutritional Cookbook, Foods, Meal Plan And Recipes for Transformative Weight Loss

DR. ALVIN BRANTLEY

Disclaimer

The information provided in this book is intended for general informational purposes only. It is not a substitute for professional medical advice, diagnosis, or treatment.

You should not use the information in this book for diagnosing or treating a health problem or disease by self decision. Always seek the advice of your physician or other qualified health provider with any questions you may have regarding a medical condition.

The author and publisher of this book make no representations or warranties with respect to the accuracy, applicability, fitness, or completeness of the contents of this book. The information contained in this book is based on the author's research and experience, and it is shared with the understanding that the author is not engaged in rendering medical, health, or any other kind of professional advice for you by this book.

The author does not endorse or promote any specific products, brands, or companies related to the contents provided in this book.

Any mention of products or services in this book is for informational purposes only and does not constitute an endorsement.

The author has not entered into any affiliate marketing agreements and has not signed any endorsement deals with individuals, organizations, or companies.

Readers are encouraged to consult with their healthcare providers before making any dietary or lifestyle chaSnges based on the information provided in this book. The author and publisher disclaim any liability for the decisions made by readers based on the information in this book.

Contents

THE TECHNIQUE UNDERLYING HCG

As a quick weight loss solution, the Human Chorionic Gonadotropin (HCG) diet has grown in popularity. The main idea behind this diet is to employ the hormone HCG, which is produced during pregnancy, to help with weight loss. For people thinking about using this diet strategy, it is imperative to comprehend the science underlying HCG.

Describe HCG.

The hormone known as HCG, or human chorionic gonadotropin, is secreted by the placenta during gestation. Its major functions are to preserve the uterine lining and aid in the growth of the fetus. It's also thought that the hormone controls how the metabolism works. Within the framework of the HCG diet, oral supplements or injections containing tiny doses of HCG are used to promote weight loss.

The Impact of HCG on Weight Loss

The idea behind the HCG diet is that HCG can aid in resetting the body's metabolism and encouraging fat loss. Dietary advocates assert that HCG can target stored fat and turn it into energy, especially in troublesome areas like the belly, thighs, and hips. To maximize the fat-burning effects of HCG, a low-calorie meal plan—often as low as 500 calories per day—is usually followed by the diet. Proponents claim that this combo causes quick weight loss without compromising muscular mass.

Critics counter that rather than the hormone's effects, the extremely low-calorie intake may be the main cause of the weight reduction seen in people following the HCG diet. They express concern about the possible hazards connected to such a restrictive diet and stress the need for a sustainable and balanced approach to weight management.

Studies & Research in Favor of HCG

There is little scientific data on the long-term safety and effectiveness of the HCG diet, despite some anecdotal evidence to the contrary. Positive results from certain research imply that HCG might help with weight loss and fat redistribution. The lack of extensive, carefully planned clinical trials and methodological errors in some of these investigations, however, cast doubt on the validity of the results.

The benefits of the HCG diet continue to divide the medical community, with groups like the Food and Drug Administration (FDA) voicing doubt and caution. A person thinking about starting an HCG diet should speak with a doctor before starting one because there are health hazards involved and there isn't enough solid research to support the diet.

The HCG diet's scientific basis is using a pregnancy-related hormone to encourage weight loss. HCG supporters contend that the hormone can specifically target stored fat and restart metabolism; however, detractors contest this claim and stress the significance of a well-rounded weight loss strategy. Because the evidence for the HCG diet is conflicting, it is advisable to proceed cautiously and get medical advice before starting any kind of plan.

CHAPTER ONE

COMMENCEMENT OF THE HCG DIET

Starting the HCG diet is a big step in the right direction for quick weight loss. It's essential to comprehend the fundamentals of the HCG diet and how it functions before getting into the specifics. At the center of this diet is the hormone HCG (human chorionic gonadotropin), which is essential for reducing appetite and promoting the body's ability to use fat reserves as fuel.

To improve weight loss outcomes, a low-calorie meal plan is frequently used with this diet.

Getting Ready For The HCG Diet Experience

Success with the HCG diet depends on preparation. It entails a thorough assessment of your eating patterns, general health, and way of living right now. Speak with a healthcare provider before beginning the diet to be sure it's a healthy choice for you.

Think about any underlying medical issues, prescription drugs, or food allergies that might affect your ability to adhere to the diet. Furthermore, because the HCG diet necessitates self-control and dedication, it is imperative to psychologically prepare for the difficulties of a low-calorie plan.

Selecting Appropriate Hcg Products

A crucial part of the HCG diet experience is choosing the appropriate HCG products. HCG comes in several forms, such as injections, drops, and pellets. Everyone has benefits and things to consider.

Because they absorb quickly, injections are a popular option, but drops and pellets are more convenient. To guarantee HCG's efficacy and safety, select a premium, pharmaceutical-grade supplement from a reliable supplier. You can choose the best option for your needs by speaking with a skilled HCG provider or a healthcare expert.

Having Reasonable Expectations

When starting the HCG diet, it's important to have reasonable expectations. While losing weight quickly is the main objective, long-term success depends on knowing the constraints and probable difficulties.

An extremely low-calorie intake is a common component of the HCG diet, which may cause immediate weight loss. But it's important to understand that everyone will respond differently to a diet and that continuing a healthy lifestyle after stopping a diet is key to avoiding weight gain.

During the diet, be ready for mood and energy swings, but keep your eyes on the goal of leading a healthy lifestyle in general.

In summary, starting the HCG diet needs careful planning and preparation.

A successful HCG journey entails knowing the basics of the diet, getting ready physically and emotionally, choosing the appropriate HCG products, and having reasonable expectations. Before beginning any weight loss program, be sure it is in line with your unique health needs and objectives by speaking with medical professionals.

CHAPTER TWO

The Hcg Diet Guidelines

The HCG (human chorionic gonadotropin) diet is a weight-loss strategy that includes supplementing with HCG hormone and following a low-calorie diet. This procedure is broken down into four separate phases, each of which has a unique function in the process of losing weight overall.

Phase 1: Days Of Loading

The loading days are the term used to describe the initial stage of the HCG diet. People are advised to begin HCG treatment with a high-calorie diet for around two days during this initial phase. This stage allows the person to accumulate fat stores while also preparing the body for the next low-calorie phase.

It is recommended that during the loading days, participants overindulge in foods high in healthy fats and carbs. The future phases of the diet will focus on releasing the aberrant fat reserves that are triggered by this brief increase in calorie intake.

Phase 2: HCG And A Low-Calorie Diet

Phase 2, when participants follow a low-calorie diet while utilizing oral HCG drops or HCG injections, is the central element of the HCG diet. This stage usually lasts for a set amount of time, between 21 and

40 days, based on personal objectives and the advice of a healthcare provider.

It is thought that the HCG hormone is essential for reducing appetite and making it easier to burn fat that has been stored as fuel. It's believed that the hormonal impacts along with the restricted calorie intake (usually 500–800 calories per day) lead to quick weight loss. During this phase, participants are advised to concentrate on eating lean proteins, vegetables, and a small amount of fruits.

Phase Three: Leveling Off

Participants go into the stability phase after the low-calorie phase, which is important to avoid rapid weight gain.

People avoid carbs and sugars and progressively raise their calorie intake during this time. Usually, this stage lasts for three weeks.

Resetting the body's metabolism and creating a new weight set point require stabilization. To keep the body from turning more calories into fat, participants keep abstaining from sugar and carbs. An important part of this phase is keeping an eye on weight swings and modifying the diet accordingly.

Phase Four: Upkeep

The maintenance phase, which comes at the end of the HCG diet, is all about switching to a longer-term, more sustainable eating schedule. Participants gradually reintegrate a greater range of items into their diets throughout this phase, all the while keeping a balanced intake.

It is critical to keep an eye on weight and modify the diet as necessary. Preventing the rebound effect and assisting people in maintaining their weight loss gains over an extended period are the objectives of the maintenance phase.

Once the HCG procedure is completed, maintaining a healthy lifestyle becomes more dependent on engaging in regular exercise and eating a nutritious, well-balanced diet.

CHAPTER THREE

Approved Meals And Plans For Eating

Because it promises quick weight loss, the Human Chorionic Gonadotropin (HCG) diet has become more and more popular. This diet combines the use of HCG hormone supplements—usually in the form of injections or oral drops—with extremely low-calorie consumption. Despite being debatable, some people report notable success with weight loss when following the HCG diet. A key component of this diet is following meal plans that are planned for each phase and sticking to a specified list of approved items.

Foods Suitable For The HCG Diet

The HCG diet places a strong emphasis on consuming particular foods that are thought to be in line with each phase's weight loss objectives.

Usually low in calories, these meals are high in nutrients that promote general health. Lean meats like turkey, chicken, and fish are acceptable sources of protein, while veggies like spinach, lettuce, and tomatoes are recommended.

Fruits including grapefruits, apples, and strawberries are also on the list, but only in small amounts. Furthermore, limited amounts of carbs from foods like whole grains are permitted. Drinking water, tea, and coffee are generally OK, and staying hydrated is important.

Sample Menus For Every Stage

Adherents of the HCG diet follow a planned regimen that changes through several phases to enhance its effectiveness. Phases one through three of the diet typically consist of loading, weight reduction, and maintenance. People are urged to eat foods high in calories during the loading period to increase their fat reserves.

A substantial calorie restriction—often as low as 500 calories per day—combined with HCG treatment characterizes the weight loss phase. During this period, sample meal plans could consist of a small quantity of fruit, a serving of vegetables, and a lean protein at each meal. To avoid weight gain, a greater range of foods is progressively added back during the maintenance phase while calorie consumption is closely monitored.

Advice For Effective Meal Planning

Efficient meal planning is crucial to following the HCG diet successfully. A crucial piece of advice is to go through and comprehend the list of foods that are permitted for each period.

Making meal plans in advance guarantees a balanced diet of fruits, vegetables, and proteins while also assisting people in staying under the recommended calorie ranges. To avoid boredom and improve dietary consumption, variety is essential.

Furthermore, cooking techniques like grilling or steaming that preserve food's nutritious content are advised.

It's critical to pay attention to serving amounts and refrain from straying from the list of permitted foods.

To keep an eye on general health and make sure the diet is both safe and appropriate for each person's needs, it is also advisable to have regular conversations with a healthcare provider.

The combination of calorie restriction, HCG supplementation, and careful adherence to meal selections is frequently credited with the success of the HCG diet. Meal plans that are well-organized and include approved meals are essential to reaching the intended weight loss goals. While some people may get quick benefits from the HCG diet, it's crucial to use caution and seek medical advice before beginning the diet to guarantee safety and efficacy.

CHAPTER FOUR

Cooking Tips And Recipes For The Hcg Diet

The human chorionic gonadotropin, or HCG, diet has become well-known because of its guarantee of quick weight loss. The diet includes consuming a few calories and administering HCG hormone by injections, drops, or pellets.

Although there is disagreement in the medical world regarding the efficacy of the HCG diet, some people have reported losing a significant amount of weight.

The selection of dishes and cooking techniques is just as important to the diet's success as calorie restriction and HCG administration.

Tasty Recipes For Every Stage

The HCG diet's phased, planned methodology is one of its main features. There are certain dietary requirements for each phase, which must be followed for the best outcomes.

It's important to include excellent dishes that follow the instructions for each phase to make the journey even more enjoyable. Focusing on nutrient-dense and filling foods during the first phase of the diet, which entails a sharp drop in calories, can help ease hunger sensations and ensure diet compliance.

Adding more recipes to the menu to vary things is crucial as the diet goes on and calorie intake goes up a little. Meals can be made more palatable and nutritious by combining fruits, vegetables, and lean proteins in interesting ways. For instance, you can stick to the diet's principles and make it more pleasant by serving grilled chicken with a colorful assortment of veggies or a refreshing fruit salad.

Cooking Techniques To Increase Nutrition And Flavor

Any diet, including the HCG diet, must include cooking if it is to be successful. Eating can be made more enjoyable overall by implementing cooking techniques that optimize flavor without sacrificing nutritional value. The best cooking techniques include steaming, baking, and grilling because they require little to no additional fat and support the diet's low-calorie requirements.

Adding new spices and herbs to foods that are HCG-approved can help improve their flavor. A good cooking experience can be enhanced by the careful use of seasonings, even when the diet may restrict some ingredients. For example, sprinkling some herbs over grilled salmon or adding some spices to a stir-fried vegetable dish might offer a taste explosion without adding a lot of calories.

Changing Up Your Best Recipes

The HCG diet's stringent rules could make it difficult to incorporate some of your favorite foods. However, customized versions of well-known recipes can be enjoyed with a little imagination and adaptability. It can be quite beneficial to replace high-calorie foods with HCG-friendly substitutes, such as rice with cauliflower instead of regular rice.

It might be necessary to experiment and be open to trying new foods while modifying meals to follow the HCG diet. The objective is to construct meals that adhere to the diet's principles without compromising flavor, but some alterations could be required. People can make the HCG diet more fun and sustainable by combining a range of flavors and textures, which increases the likelihood that they will succeed in losing weight in the long run.

CHAPTER FIVE

Overcoming Difficulties And Failures

Starting the HCG diet can be difficult, and there can be several challenges that people run across. Controlling hunger and cravings is one of the main difficulties, particularly because the diet is low in calories. Furthermore, it might be challenging to navigate social settings where food is the main topic. Developing solutions to get past these obstacles and continue on the path to reaching weight loss objectives is essential.

Handling Cravings And Hunger

A very low-calorie intake is a common component of the HCG diet, which may increase cravings and sensations of hunger. Drinking plenty of water and eating foods that are permitted on the diet are crucial for reducing unpleasant feelings. Lean proteins and foods high in fiber might help you feel fuller for longer. Furthermore, dividing meals into smaller, more regular servings throughout the day may aid in better-controlling hunger.

To deal with cravings, it's a good idea to investigate fun and HCG diet-compliant dishes. A more sustainable diet can be achieved by substituting favorite snacks or sweets from the authorized food list. Moreover, mindful eating techniques and the ability to distinguish between actual hunger and emotional cravings might enable people to make better decisions while on the HCG journey.

Handling Social Circumstances

Following the HCG diet's restrictions can make it difficult to attend social events or get-togethers. Making the hosts aware of any dietary needs or bringing foods that fit the requirements to share can help guarantee that there are appropriate options available.

Making a plan and having a modest but filling meal before going to social gatherings can also help reduce the desire to stray from the diet. Furthermore, in these circumstances, it might be quite important to ask friends and family for support, since their understanding and encouragement can help one stick to the HCG diet.

Typical Mistakes And How To Prevent Them

The HCG diet has drawbacks despite its possible advantages. One frequent error that can undermine the efficacy of a diet is giving in to the urge to stray from the approved food list.

It is crucial to comprehend the permitted foods in great detail and to follow the instructions in the letter.

Furthermore, there could be hazards or consequences to your health if you begin the HCG diet without first consulting a doctor. To guarantee the diet is secure and appropriate for each person's needs, routine examinations and monitoring are essential.

Relying too much on HCG supplements without appropriate supervision is another risk to be aware of.

To prevent any negative consequences, HCG should only be used under the supervision of a licensed healthcare provider.

Also, if long-term lifestyle adjustments are not made, people may have a rebound effect after finishing the diet and rapidly acquire weight again.

After the HCG phase is over, it's critical to switch to a nutritious, balanced diet and engage in regular exercise to avoid this.

Even while the HCG diet may promote quick weight loss, a successful and long-lasting result depends on overcoming obstacles and avoiding typical errors. People can better manage the HCG diet and increase their chances of reaching their targeted weight loss objectives by addressing concerns with hunger, cravings, and social circumstances.

CHAPTER SIX

Hcg Interaction With Exercise:

Those looking to improve their weight reduction journey may be interested in learning more about how to incorporate exercise into the HCG diet plan. Exercise, according to several supporters, can enhance energy expenditure, speed up metabolism, and enhance general well-being, all of which can enhance the benefits of HCG supplementation.

Exercise's Place In The HCG Diet:

A variety of factors influence exercise on the HCG diet. Supporters of this strategy claim that including exercise can help retain muscle mass, preventing the loss of muscle that is frequently linked to low-calorie diets. Additionally, by encouraging fat burning and raising metabolic efficiency, exercise may help to promote a more sustainable and balanced weight loss.

Safe And Efficient Exercise Programs At Every Stage:

When adding exercise, it's important to know what the demands are for each stage of the HCG diet.

During the first stage, which is marked by an extremely low-calorie diet, concentrate on low- to moderate-intensity physical activities like swimming, yoga, or brisk walking.

More rigorous exercises like strength training and high-intensity interval training (HIIT) can be gradually added as the diet improves and calorie intake rises.

A wider variety of exercises can be included when the calorie intake normalizes throughout the maintenance period.

A more varied exercise program, incorporating aerobic, weight training, and flexibility exercises, is possible at this phase.

To prevent overexertion, it is crucial to adjust the intensity of the workout to each person's degree of fitness and pay attention to your body's cues.

Managing Physical Activity And Quick Weight Loss:

To avoid detrimental health impacts, striking a balance between activity and fast weight loss is essential. Before starting an exercise program, it is imperative to speak with a healthcare provider or fitness specialist, particularly if you're on a low-calorie diet like HCG. Maintaining a good balance requires keeping an eye on energy levels, modifying the intensity of workouts accordingly, and making sure you're getting enough nutrition and fluids.

Exercise can provide benefits beyond calorie restriction and hormone supplementation, which are the main goals of the HCG diet.

A more comprehensive and long-lasting approach to quick weight loss may involve combining HCG with exercise, which can improve overall well-being and preserve muscle mass.

Personalized coaching and exercise of caution are necessary to achieve the proper balance and guarantee the security and efficacy of this combination strategy.

CHAPTER SEVEN

Hcg Diet Success Stories

The HCG (Human Chorionic Gonadotropin) diet has gained popularity for its claim to facilitate rapid weight loss. Many individuals embark on this diet journey with the hope of achieving significant results in a short period. Exploring real-life success stories provides insight into the effectiveness of the HCG diet and the transformative experiences of those who have embraced it.

Real-Life Experiences Of Individuals On The HCG Diet

One common theme among HCG diet success stories is the rapidity of weight loss. Individuals often report shedding pounds at an accelerated pace compared to traditional dieting methods.

These real-life accounts highlight the tangible impact of the HCG hormone in conjunction with a low-calorie diet. Many express their initial skepticism but are ultimately amazed at the visible changes in their body composition.

Participants in the HCG diet often underscore the importance of strict adherence to the prescribed protocol. Following the recommended caloric intake and incorporating the HCG hormone effectively are pivotal factors in achieving the desired results. These personal narratives emphasize the significance of commitment and discipline throughout the diet, showcasing the transformative power of the HCG protocol when implemented correctly.

Lessons Learned And Tips For Success

Within the realm of HCG diet success stories, certain common lessons emerge. Participants frequently share insights into overcoming challenges and maintaining motivation during the process.

Learning to navigate social situations and resist temptations is a recurring theme, emphasizing the importance of mental resilience.

Many individuals stress the need for a strong support system, whether it be friends, family, or online communities, to share experiences and seek guidance.

Tips for success often revolve around meal planning, creativity in food choices, and finding alternatives to high-calorie ingredients.

Participants stress the significance of staying hydrated and incorporating light exercise to enhance the weight loss process.

Additionally, they highlight the importance of consulting healthcare professionals before starting the HCG diet to ensure its safety and appropriateness for individual health conditions.

In conclusion, the HCG diet success stories provide a compelling narrative of rapid weight loss and personal transformation.

These accounts offer valuable insights into the challenges and triumphs associated with the HCG diet, shedding light on the importance of commitment, discipline, and a supportive environment in achieving successful outcomes.

CHAPTER EIGHT

Beyond The Hcg Diet

The Human Chorionic Gonadotropin (HCG) diet has gained popularity as a rapid weight loss method, primarily due to its promise of shedding pounds quickly. While the HCG diet can be effective in the short term, it is essential to consider the post-diet phase to ensure sustainable weight management.

Maintaining Weight Loss After HCG

Once you've completed the HCG diet and achieved your desired weight loss, the challenge lies in maintaining those results. One key aspect is gradually transitioning back to a more conventional and sustainable eating pattern. It's crucial to understand that the strict caloric restrictions imposed during the HCG phase are not viable for the long term.

Maintaining weight loss involves finding a balance between calorie intake and expenditure. Implementing a well-rounded and nutritionally balanced diet is vital. Focus on incorporating a variety of nutrient-dense foods, including lean proteins, whole grains, fruits, and vegetables. Portion control and mindful eating play significant roles in preventing weight regain.

Regular physical activity remains a cornerstone for maintaining weight loss. Engaging in a mix of aerobic exercises, strength training, and flexibility exercises contributes to overall well-being. Establishing a consistent exercise routine helps burn calories, build lean muscle mass, and boost metabolism, all of which are instrumental in sustaining weight loss.

Developing Healthy Habits For Long-Term Success

Beyond the immediate focus on weight loss, developing and maintaining healthy habits is essential for long-term success. Rather than relying solely on the restrictive nature of the HCG diet, consider incorporating sustainable habits into your daily life.

This includes adopting a balanced and varied diet, staying hydrated, and getting sufficient sleep.

Cultivating a mindful approach to eating is crucial. Pay attention to hunger and fullness cues, and avoid emotional or stress-related eating.

Building a positive relationship with food involves savoring meals, making mindful food choices, and addressing underlying issues that may contribute to unhealthy eating habits.

Regular monitoring of weight and health markers is a proactive approach. Periodic check-ins with a healthcare professional can provide guidance and support in maintaining optimal health. Adjustments to dietary and lifestyle habits may be necessary over time, and a healthcare provider can offer personalized advice based on individual needs and goals.

Exploring Continued Health And Wellness

While the HCG diet may kick-start weight loss, it's important to view health and wellness holistically.

Beyond just focusing on the number on the scale, consider other aspects of well-being, such as mental health, stress management, and overall lifestyle. Sustainable health is a dynamic and ongoing process that involves continuous self-care.

Explore additional wellness strategies, such as mindfulness practices, stress reduction techniques, and adequate self-care.

These elements contribute to a comprehensive approach to health, addressing not only physical but also mental and emotional well-being. Building a foundation of overall wellness ensures that weight management becomes a part of a broader commitment to a healthy and fulfilling life.

Conclusion

In conclusion, the HCG diet has become a popular choice for those seeking rapid weight loss. While some individuals report success and improved well-being, the diet is not without controversy and challenges. The role of HCG in the weight loss process remains a topic of debate within the medical community, and potential risks should be carefully considered. As with any weight loss strategy, consulting with healthcare professionals is essential to make informed decisions about one's health.

Celebrating Your Hcg Diet Journey

Embarking on the HCG diet is a significant commitment to one's health and well-being. Celebrate the milestones, both big and small, throughout your weight loss journey. Recognize the efforts you put into making positive lifestyle changes and achieving your goals. Whether it's fitting into smaller clothing or experiencing improved energy levels, take pride in your accomplishments and use them as motivation to continue on your path to a healthier you.

Looking Ahead To A Healthier Future

As you wrap up your HCG diet journey, it's essential to shift your focus to maintaining a healthy lifestyle. Establish sustainable habits, including balanced nutrition, regular physical activity, and mindful eating. Set realistic and achievable goals for long-term wellness. Remember that a healthy lifestyle is a continuous journey, and by staying committed to your well-being, you can enjoy the benefits of improved health and vitality for years to come.